GENITAL HERPES

PRACTICAL TACTIS FOR HEALING GENITAL HERPES

DR. J. WALLER

1

Contents

Introduction

Genital herpes is a common sexually transmitted infection (STI) caused by the herpes simplex virus (HSV). The virus primarily spreads through sexual contact and can affect the genital, anal, and surrounding areas. There are two main types of herpes simplex virus: HSV-1 and HSV-2. While HSV-1 is traditionally associated with oral herpes (cold sores), either type can cause genital herpes.

Genital herpes is characterized by the development of painful sores or blisters in the genital and anal regions. These outbreaks can be recurrent, with periods of symptom-free intervals in between. In addition to physical symptoms, genital herpes can also have emotional and psychological impacts due to the stigma associated with STIs.

Prevention measures include practicing safe sex, using condoms, and open communication with sexual partners. Although there is no cure for genital herpes, antiviral medications can help manage symptoms and reduce the frequency of outbreaks.

It's important for individuals with genital herpes to seek medical advice, adhere to prescribed treatments, and engage in open discussions with healthcare providers and sexual partners for effective management and support.

CHAPTER ONE

Understanding Genital Herpes

Genital herpes is a sexually transmitted infection (STI) caused by the herpes simplex virus (HSV), primarily HSV-1 or HSV-2. Here's a deeper understanding of genital herpes:

Transmission:

Genital herpes spreads through direct skin-to-skin contact with an infected person during sexual activities. It can be transmitted through vaginal, anal, or oral sex, even when the infected person is not experiencing visible symptoms.

Two Types of Herpes Simplex Virus:

HSV-1: Typically associated with oral herpes (cold sores), but can also cause genital herpes through oral-genital contact.

HSV-2: Mainly associated with genital herpes. However, both HSV-1 and HSV-2 can cause infections in either location.

Symptoms:

Genital herpes often presents with painful sores or blisters in the genital or anal area. Other symptoms may include itching, burning sensations, and flu-like symptoms such as fever and swollen lymph nodes.

Recurrence:

After the initial infection, the virus remains in the body and can cause recurrent outbreaks. The frequency and severity of outbreaks vary among individuals.

Asymptomatic Shedding:

Even when no visible symptoms are present, individuals with genital herpes can still shed the virus and potentially transmit it to sexual partners.

Diagnosis:

Diagnosis is typically based on clinical symptoms, medical history, and laboratory tests, such as PCR (polymerase chain reaction) or viral culture from a swab of the affected area.

Management and Treatment:

While there is no cure for genital herpes, antiviral medications such as acyclovir, valacyclovir, and famciclovir can help manage symptoms, reduce the frequency of outbreaks, and lower the risk of transmission.

Prevention:

Safe Sex: Consistent and correct use of condoms during sexual activity can reduce the risk of transmission.

Communication: Open and honest communication with sexual partners about STI status is crucial for preventing transmission.

Antiviral Medications: Taking antiviral medications as prescribed can reduce the risk of transmission to partners.

Psychosocial Impact:

Living with genital herpes may have emotional and psychological implications due to stigma and misconceptions. Support from healthcare professionals, counselors, and support groups can be beneficial.

Pregnancy and Genital Herpes:

Pregnant individuals with genital herpes should inform their healthcare providers. While the risk of transmission to the baby is low, it can have severe consequences if transmission occurs during childbirth.

It's important for individuals with genital herpes to seek medical advice, practice safe sex, and communicate openly with sexual partners.

Regular medical check-ups and ongoing support contribute to effective management and a better quality of life.

The asymptomatic nature of genital herpes

Genital herpes can have an asymptomatic or minimally symptomatic nature, meaning that individuals infected with the herpes simplex virus (HSV) may not experience noticeable signs or symptoms. This aspect of genital herpes adds complexity to its diagnosis and management. Here are key points regarding the asymptomatic nature of genital herpes:

Subclinical Infections:

Some individuals infected with HSV, particularly HSV-2, may remain asymptomatic throughout their lives. These individuals carry the virus but do not develop visible sores or experience the typical symptoms associated with genital herpes.

Asymptomatic Shedding:

Even in the absence of visible symptoms, individuals with genital herpes can shed the virus and potentially transmit it to sexual partners. This is known as asymptomatic shedding and occurs periodically.

Transmission Risk:

Asymptomatic shedding poses a risk of transmission to sexual partners, and the risk is not eliminated by the absence of visible symptoms. Condom use and antiviral medications can help reduce the risk of transmission.

Undiagnosed Cases:

Because some individuals with genital herpes may not experience noticeable symptoms, the infection can go undiagnosed. This can contribute to the unintentional spread of the virus.

Diagnostic Challenges:

The lack of visible symptoms makes it challenging to diagnose asymptomatic cases. Laboratory tests, such as PCR (polymerase chain reaction) or viral culture from a swab of the affected area, are used to detect the virus in both symptomatic and asymptomatic individuals.

Impact on Transmission Dynamics:

The asymptomatic nature of genital herpes plays a significant role in the epidemiology of the infection. It contributes to the widespread prevalence of HSV in the population, as individuals may unknowingly transmit the virus.

Preventive Measures:

Regular Testing: Routine testing for HSV, especially in high-risk populations, can help identify asymptomatic cases.

Safe Sex Practices: Consistent and correct use of condoms, along with open communication about

STI status with sexual partners, remains crucial for preventing transmission.

Psychosocial Implications:

Asymptomatic carriers may be unaware of their infection, which can impact their psychosocial well-being if diagnosed later. Education and counseling are essential components of managing the emotional aspects of herpes infections.

Understanding the asymptomatic nature of genital herpes underscores the importance of routine testing, communication about STI status, and preventive measures to reduce the risk of transmission. Individuals with concerns about genital herpes or their sexual health should consult with healthcare professionals for guidance and appropriate testing.

Genital herpes symptoms can vary from person to person, and some individuals may experience asymptomatic infections. When symptoms do occur, they typically manifest as follows:

Painful Sores or Blisters:

Small, painful sores or blisters may appear in the genital or anal areas. These lesions can break open and form ulcers before healing.

Stitching and Sensitivity:

The affected area may be itchy and irritated, contributing to discomfort.

CHAPTER TWO

Flu-Like Symptoms:

Some individuals may experience flu-like symptoms, including fever, headaches, muscle aches, and swollen lymph nodes during the initial outbreak.

Pain or Discomfort during Urination:

Urinating when lesions are present can cause pain or discomfort.

Vaginal Discharge (Women):

Women may experience abnormal vaginal discharge along with other symptoms.

Pain in the Lower Abdomen:

Pain or tenderness in the lower abdomen may occur, especially during the initial outbreak.

Painful Sex:

Sexual intercourse can be painful due to the presence of sores and lesions.

It's important to note that symptoms can vary in severity, and some individuals may have mild or atypical presentations. Additionally, recurrent outbreaks may have fewer symptoms than the initial outbreak.

In cases of asymptomatic infections, individuals may not experience noticeable signs or symptoms. However, even in the absence of visible symptoms, the virus can still be shed, posing a risk of transmission to sexual partners.

If you suspect you have genital herpes or experience symptoms consistent with the infection, it's crucial to seek prompt medical attention for an accurate diagnosis and appropriate management. Testing for herpes simplex virus (HSV) through laboratory methods, such as PCR (polymerase chain reaction) or viral culture, can help confirm the diagnosis.

Transmission Realities

The transmission of genital herpes involves the spread of the herpes simplex virus (HSV) through direct skin-to-skin contact. Here are the key transmission realities of genital herpes:

Sexual Contact:

Genital herpes is primarily transmitted through sexual activities involving the exchange of genital, anal, or oral fluids. This includes vaginal, anal, and oral sex.

Virus Shedding:

Individuals with genital herpes can shed the virus even when they are not experiencing visible symptoms (asymptomatic shedding). Asymptomatic shedding contributes to the risk of transmission to sexual partners.

Presence of Sores or Lesions:

The risk of transmission is highest when visible symptoms, such as sores or lesions, are present. These areas of active infection contain a high concentration of the virus.

Asymptomatic Transmission:

Asymptomatic carriers, who do not have visible symptoms, can still transmit the virus to sexual partners. The risk is not eliminated by the absence of noticeable sores.

Use of Condoms:

Consistent and correct use of condoms during sexual activities can reduce the risk of transmission. However, condoms do not provide complete protection, as they may not cover all potentially infectious areas.

Antiviral Medications:

Taking antiviral medications, such as acyclovir, valacyclovir, or famciclovir, can help reduce the frequency of outbreaks and lower the risk of transmission. These medications are often prescribed for both symptomatic and asymptomatic individuals.

Prevention Through Communication:

Open communication between sexual partners about their sexual health, including STI status, is crucial for preventing transmission. This allows for informed decision-making and joint efforts to reduce risk.

Avoidance during Outbreaks:

Sexual activities should be avoided during outbreaks when sores or lesions are present, as this is when the risk of transmission is highest.

Pregnancy and Transmission:

Pregnant individuals with genital herpes should inform their healthcare providers. While the risk of transmission to the baby is low, precautions may be taken to minimize the risk during childbirth.

Understanding the realities of genital herpes transmission emphasizes the importance of safe sex practices, open communication, and medical management. Regular testing, particularly in high-risk populations, can help identify and address infections, contributing to the prevention of transmission. Individuals with concerns about genital herpes or their sexual health should consult with healthcare professionals for guidance and appropriate testing.

The diagnosis and testing of genital herpes involve a combination of clinical assessment, laboratory tests, and, in some cases, imaging studies. Here's an overview of the methods used for the diagnosis of genital herpes:

Clinical Evaluation:

Healthcare providers start with a thorough medical history and physical examination to evaluate symptoms and potential risk factors. The appearance and location of sores or lesions are crucial in the clinical assessment.

Swab Test (Viral Culture or PCR):

The most common and reliable method for diagnosing genital herpes is by taking a swab sample from an active sore or lesion. The sample is then tested using viral culture or polymerase chain reaction (PCR) to detect the presence of the herpes simplex virus (HSV).

Blood Examinations:

Blood tests, such as type-specific serology tests, can determine the presence of antibodies against HSV-1 and HSV-2. These tests are particularly useful in cases of asymptomatic or atypical presentations and can help identify previous infections.

Antigen Detection Tests:

Antigen detection tests can be used to detect viral proteins from swab samples. However, these tests are less commonly used compared to viral culture or PCR.

Biopsy:

In some cases, a biopsy of the affected tissue may be performed to confirm the diagnosis, especially if the presentation is atypical.

Imaging Research:

In rare cases, imaging studies such as magnetic resonance imaging (MRI) may be used to assess complications or involvement of deeper tissues.

It's important to note that the timing of testing is crucial. For swab tests, it's best to collect samples during the early stages of an outbreak when sores or lesions are present. Blood tests can be conducted at any time, but they may not provide accurate results immediately after infection, and they may not differentiate between recent and past infections.

Genital herpes testing is recommended for individuals experiencing symptoms consistent with the infection, those with a known exposure to the virus, and those seeking routine STI screening. Open communication with healthcare providers about symptoms and sexual history is essential for accurate diagnosis and appropriate management.

The management of genital herpes involves antiviral medications to reduce symptoms, control outbreaks, and lower the risk of transmission. Here are the key treatment approaches for genital herpes:

Antiviral Medications:

Acyclovir: Available in oral, intravenous, and topical forms, acyclovir is one of the first-line medications for genital herpes. It helps reduce the severity and duration of outbreaks.

Valacyclovir: This prodrug of acyclovir is converted to acyclovir in the body and has similar efficacy. Valacyclovir is often preferred due to its more convenient dosing regimen.

Famciclovir: Another antiviral medication that is effective in managing genital herpes. It is taken orally and helps control symptoms and outbreaks.

Episodic Treatment:

Episodic treatment involves taking antiviral medications at the onset of symptoms or during outbreaks to shorten the duration and alleviate symptoms.

Suppressive Treatment:

Suppressive or daily therapy involves taking antiviral medications on a daily basis, regardless of symptoms. This approach is recommended for individuals with frequent or severe outbreaks and aims to reduce the frequency of recurrences and lower the risk of transmission.

Initiation of Treatment during Initial Outbreak:

Antiviral medications are often initiated during the initial outbreak to accelerate healing, reduce symptoms, and potentially decrease the severity of subsequent outbreaks.

Management of Asymptomatic Shedding:

Daily antiviral therapy is effective in reducing asymptomatic shedding, lowering the risk of transmission to sexual partners.

Pregnancy Management:

Pregnant individuals with genital herpes may be prescribed antiviral medications to reduce the risk of transmission to the baby during childbirth. It's essential to discuss treatment options and potential risks with healthcare providers during pregnancy.

Pain Management:

Over-the-counter pain relievers, such as acetaminophen or ibuprofen, may be recommended to alleviate pain and discomfort associated with outbreaks.

Topical Interventions:

Topical antiviral creams may be prescribed for localized lesions, but they are generally less effective than oral antiviral medications.

It's important for individuals with genital herpes to consult with healthcare providers for personalized treatment plans based on the frequency and severity of outbreaks, individual health considerations, and the potential impact on sexual partners. While antiviral medications can help manage symptoms and reduce the risk of transmission, there is no cure for genital herpes. Education about the condition, counseling, and support play crucial roles in the holistic management of genital herpes.

Living with Genital Herpes

Living with genital herpes involves managing the physical symptoms, navigating emotional aspects, and taking steps to reduce the risk of transmission. Here are key aspects of living with genital herpes:

Medical Management:

Antiviral Medications: Consistent use of antiviral medications, either episodically or as suppressive therapy, can help manage symptoms, reduce the frequency of outbreaks, and lower the risk of transmission.

Regular Check-ups: Periodic medical check-ups are essential to monitor the effectiveness of treatment, assess overall health, and address any concerns.

Symptom Management:

Pain Relief: Over-the-counter pain relievers can help alleviate pain and discomfort during outbreaks.

Topical Treatments: For localized lesions, topical antiviral creams may be prescribed.

Psychosocial Support:

Counseling: Seeking counseling or therapy can provide emotional support and help individuals cope with the psychological impact of genital herpes.

Support Groups: Joining support groups or online communities allows individuals to connect with others facing similar challenges, share experiences, and gain valuable insights.

CHAPTER THREE

Disclosure and Communication:

Open Communication: Transparent communication with sexual partners about one's STI status, including genital herpes, is crucial. This allows partners to make informed decisions about their sexual health.

Disclosure Strategies: Deciding when and how to disclose one's status can vary. Some individuals choose to disclose early in a relationship, while others may wait until they feel more comfortable.

Safe Sex Practices:

Condom Use: Consistent and correct use of condoms during sexual activities helps reduce the risk of transmission, although it does not eliminate it entirely.

Suppressive Therapy: For individuals in relationships with uninfected partners, suppressive antiviral therapy can further lower the risk of transmission.

Pregnancy Considerations:

Medical Guidance: Pregnant individuals with genital herpes should inform their healthcare providers. Medical guidance and precautions may be provided to minimize the risk of transmission to the baby during childbirth.

Regular Testing:

Regular testing for other sexually transmitted infections (STIs) is important to maintain overall sexual health.

Wellness Practices:

Adopting a healthy lifestyle, including regular exercise, a balanced diet, and stress management, contributes to overall well-being.

Resources for Education:

Staying informed about genital herpes, transmission realities, and treatment options empowers individuals to make informed decisions about their health.

Living with genital herpes may pose challenges, but with proper medical management, support, and communication, individuals can lead fulfilling lives. Seeking professional guidance, staying connected with supportive communities, and prioritizing overall well-being contribute to effective management and a positive outlook.

Preventive Strategies

Preventive strategies for genital herpes aim to reduce the risk of transmission and minimize the frequency and severity of outbreaks. Here are key preventive measures:

Safe Sex Practices:

Condom Use: Consistent and correct use of latex or polyurethane condoms during sexual activities can help reduce the risk of transmission. While condoms do not provide complete protection, they offer a level of barrier against genital herpes.

Antiviral Medications:

Suppressive Therapy: Taking antiviral medications on a daily basis as suppressive therapy can significantly lower the risk of transmission to sexual partners. This approach is particularly beneficial for individuals with frequent or severe outbreaks.

Regular Testing:

Regular testing for genital herpes and other sexually transmitted infections (STIs) is crucial, especially for individuals with multiple sexual partners or those in new relationships. Early detection allows for prompt treatment and preventive measures.

Communication and Disclosure:

Open Communication: Honest and open communication with sexual partners about one's STI status, including genital herpes, is essential. Partners can make informed decisions about their sexual health and risk tolerance.

Avoidance during Outbreaks:

Refraining from sexual activities during outbreaks when sores or lesions are present can minimize the risk of transmission.

Counseling and Education:

Seeking counseling or education about genital herpes, transmission risks, and preventive strategies can provide individuals with the knowledge and tools to make informed decisions about their sexual health.

Pregnancy Planning:

Pregnant individuals with genital herpes should discuss their condition with healthcare providers to develop a plan for managing the risk of transmission to the baby during childbirth.

Regular Medical Check-ups:

Regular check-ups with healthcare providers allow for monitoring of overall health, adjustment of treatment plans, and addressing any concerns related to genital herpes.

Handling Stress:

Stress can trigger outbreaks, so adopting stress management techniques, such as exercise, relaxation, and mindfulness, may help reduce the frequency of outbreaks.

Partner Screening:

Encouraging sexual partners to undergo testing for STIs, including genital herpes, is a proactive step in preventing transmission. Knowing each other's status allows for joint decision-making about preventive measures.

It's important to note that while these strategies can reduce the risk of transmission, they do not eliminate it entirely. No method offers 100% protection. Individuals with genital herpes should work closely with healthcare providers to develop a comprehensive preventive plan tailored to their specific needs and circumstances. Additionally, staying informed about the latest developments in herpes research and treatment options contributes to effective prevention.

CONCLUSION

In conclusion, genital herpes is a common sexually transmitted infection caused by the herpes simplex virus (HSV). Living with genital herpes involves managing physical symptoms, navigating emotional aspects, and adopting preventive strategies to reduce the risk of transmission.

Key items to consider:

Medical Management: Antiviral medications play a crucial role in managing symptoms, controlling outbreaks, and lowering the risk of transmission. Episodic or suppressive therapy may be recommended based on individual needs.

Symptom Management: Over-the-counter pain relievers and topical treatments can help alleviate pain and discomfort during outbreaks.

Psychosocial Support: Counseling, support groups, and online communities offer valuable emotional support for individuals living with genital herpes.

Disclosure and Communication: Open communication with sexual partners about one's

STI status is essential for informed decision-making and prevention.

Safe Sex Practices: Consistent condom use, suppressive therapy, and avoidance of sexual activities during outbreaks contribute to preventive measures.

Regular Testing: Routine testing for genital herpes and other STIs is crucial for early detection, prompt treatment, and prevention.

Pregnancy Considerations: Pregnant individuals with genital herpes should work with healthcare providers to manage the risk of transmission to the baby during childbirth.

Wellness Practices: Adopting a healthy lifestyle, including regular exercise, a balanced diet, and stress management, contributes to overall well-being.

While there is no cure for genital herpes, education, counseling, and support enable individuals to lead fulfilling lives. With proactive management and preventive strategies, the impact of genital herpes on both physical and emotional well-being can be minimized. Seeking professional guidance, staying informed, and fostering open communication contribute to a positive outlook for individuals living with genital herpes.

THE END

www.ingramcontent.com/pod-product-compliance
Lightning Source LLC
Chambersburg PA
CBHW060816260726
48660CB00002B/981